THE
Sleep Guide

Tips and Tricks for a Better Night's Sleep

Mark Richardson

It's Time to Get the Sleep You Deserve

It's 2am and you're wide awake. You're staring at the ceiling, feeling increasingly anxious as the minutes tick by. Your mind focuses on all the sleep you're missing out on with each passing hour.

You probably have a full list of reasons why you'd rather be sleeping right now. Maybe you need to be on top of your game for a presentation at work in the morning. Maybe your body feels exhausted, or you know you'll be sleepy and cranky all day tomorrow. Maybe you're just bored to tears from the constant tossing and turning night after night after night.

Whatever your reasons are, you're right to want to fall asleep and stay asleep. It's not too much to ask! We all deserve to sleep soundly, but for many of us, sleep slips through our fingers every night.

Insomnia and other sleeping problems are

major concerns for many more people than you might think. It's estimated that 70 million Americans have difficulty falling or staying asleep. Even if you've made time for the recommended 7-8 hours of sleep, you may be unable to take full advantage of your time in bed.

This guide was written to provide you with the information you need to sleep better. It offers you the best tips and tricks to improve the quantity and quality of your sleep each and every night. It's time to start getting the sleep you need. Reading this guide is your first step to better sleep!

Why Sleep Matters

Learning and Memory
Metabolism and Weight
Safety and Judgement
Mood

1

Support your learning and memory

If you're struggling to learn new skills, activities, or languages, or even if you're just trying to remember your grocery list, better sleep can be a powerful solution.

Our brains sift through information and make connections while we sleep. Not getting enough sleep at night can hurt our ability to use information that we've previously learned.

Think back to your school years. Staying up all night made remembering information for tests much harder.

Information doesn't sink in the first time we try to memorize or learn it. When we crammed for tests the night before, we threw all that information into our short-term memory, but didn't give our brains a chance to process it.

Our short-term memory are constantly being replaced with new information, and this information isn't committed to our long-term memory until we sleep at night.

2

Sleep for healthy metabolism and weight

When we are fatigued, we lack the energy to exercise and lose the motivation to eat right. We often try to fight fatigue by eating the nearest bag of chips or downing a quick cup of coffee. As you know, a poor diet and lack of exercise is the perfect recipe for weight gain.

Our urge to eat causes changes in our bodies' hormone levels. Sleep deprivation increases our bodies' levels of ghrelin, stimulating our appetite and making us hungrier. It also decreases our bodies' leptin levels. Leptin signals our bodies to stop eating when we're full. Lack of sleep can cause us to eat too much, adding weight to our bodies and inches to our waist lines. If you are dieting or want to maintain a healthy weight, getting plenty of sleep every night may help you reach your goals successfully!

3

Stay safe and improve judgement with sleep

Have you ever looked back at a bad decision and wondered what you were thinking at the time? Lack of sleep slows our reaction times and impairs our decision making.

Our performances in simple tasks, like driving, can also be impaired. Lack of sleep affects our bodies in a way similar to alcohol intoxication. Driving while sleep-deprived is as dangerous as driving drunk.

Getting a solid night's sleep helps you get to work safely, make sound decisions, and perform at your best.

4

Improve your mood and relationships

The amount of sleep we get each night affects our overall moods. Studies of patients with sleep deprivation show an increase in stress, anger, sadness, and mental exhaustion.

Our moods can have a major impact on our interpersonal relationships. When we are stressed and frustrated from lack of sleep, we may unintentionally take it out on those around us. We lose patience and find it difficult to enjoy activities and time with our loved ones.

Getting a good night's sleep can not only help improve our personal moods, but it can also benefit our relationships.

The Stages of Sleep

Light Sleep
Stage 2 Sleep
Deep Sleep
Rapid Eye Movement (REM) Sleep

1

Light sleep

Light sleep, the first and shortest stage of sleep, typically lasts for about 10 minutes. In this stage, your body transitions from full consciousness to deeper sleep. During this transition, you are easily woken by sound or light.

In light sleep, your brain transitions from producing fast to slow brain waves as your body slows down. Brain waves are a measure of your brain's activity level. When you are awake, your brain produces small, fast waves. When you are asleep, your brain waves are slower, with occasional bursts of rapid brain activity.

2

Stage 2 sleep

Stage 2 sleep follows light sleep and accounts for about 40-50% of your total sleep time. By Stage 2, you have lost all awareness of the world around you.

In comparison to light sleep, Stage 2 sleep is deeper. Your brain slows down even more and emits fewer fast brain waves. Your heart rate slows and your body's temperature decreases in preparation for entering deep sleep.

When you first fall asleep, you will progress from Stage 2 sleep into the deeper sleep of Stage 3. Therefore, Stage 2 is an important stage necessary to reach deeper and more refreshing sleep. Your body will cycle through the stages of sleep many times throughout the night. As a result, you will return to Stage 2 sleep several times during an average night's sleep.

3
Deep sleep

Deep sleep makes up 20% of a healthy night's sleep. During deep sleep, all eye and muscle movement ceases, and you become difficult to wake. Very slow brain waves emerge in this sleep stage.

Deep sleep is necessary to feel refreshed in the morning. If you are woken during deep sleep, you may feel groggy and disoriented for several minutes.

4

Rapid Eye Movement (REM) sleep

Rapid Eye Movement (REM) describes the physical movement of your eyes. Your mind is very active during this time, and your eyes move rapidly beneath eyelids. Despite your eye movement the rest of your body is in a state of paralysis.

REM sleep typically takes up about 90-120 minutes of a typical night's sleep over the course of four or five different periods.

Although dreams may occur in other sleep stages, vividly-recalled dreams are more likely to occur during REM sleep.

30
Tips for a Better Night's Sleep

1

Soak up the early morning sun.

Light helps us wake up in the morning. Getting sun for 20 minutes in the morning signals your brain to wake up. Early in the day is the best time to get sunlight because it resets your body's rhythms. Try getting sunlight between 6 and 8:30 am.

A great way to fit in your daily sun exposure is to walk to work (at least partway) in the morning. If your morning commute limits your sun exposure, try eating lunch outside or taking a walk around the block during your lunch break.

2

Keep the same schedule every day.

Try to wake up and go to bed at around the same time everyday. A regular schedule helps your body keep a healthy cycle.

Avoid having to catch up on sleep on the weekends. This overload can contribute to sleep disturbance.

If you have trouble waking up in the morning, one easy trick to motivate an early start time is to deliberately schedule activities or appointments earlier in the day. This will help you commit to a set schedule.

By switching to a more consistent sleep schedule, you may find that your body feels refreshed and ready to start the day!

3

Exercise regularly.

In addition to its myriad of health benefits, regular exercise can also improve your sleep.

Just as sleeping at the same time each night regulates your body's sleep cycle, exercising helps regulate your body's metabolism, allowing your body to energize during the day and refresh at night.

Try to get your heart pumping for at least 30 minutes every day, preferably in the morning. If you can't get up that early or don't have the time, try breaking up your exercise throughout the day. Split your exercise between mornings, lunchtimes, and after work.

If you exercise later in the day, aim to finish your activity at least 3 hours before your bedtime to allow your body time to wind down before sleep.

4

Nap smart.

Daytime napping can take away your ability to sleep soundly through the night. If you accidentally fall asleep in front of the TV, you could have trouble falling asleep at bedtime.

Done properly, napping can be an effective way to boost energy and productivity during the day, especially when you aren't able to get enough sleep at night.

A short "power nap" can be great for refueling your body when fatigued, but it should be limited to just 20 to 30 minutes. If you sleep longer than that, you are likely to wake up feeling more tired than you did before your nap!

Beware of untimed naps – they can turn into a long sleep that can dramatically disrupt your sleep schedule. Avoid napping after 4pm to prevent interference with your nighttime sleeping.

5

Wake up earlier.

Can't fall asleep at night? Internal clock out of sync from a crazy schedule or recent travel?

If you find yourself lying awake at night unable to sleep, try waking up 30 minutes earlier the following morning. Not only will you have more time for your morning routine, but you'll teach your body that it won't be able to get extra, catch-up sleep in the mornings.

After a few days, your sleep schedule will shift. As a result, you will begin to feel sleepier at your chosen bedtime and spend less time trying to fall asleep at night.

6

Avoid alcoholic beverages before bedtime.

Although alcohol may make you feel sleepy, you should avoid it before bed. Alcohol can disrupt the balance between REM and non-REM sleep. Alcohol makes the time you spend sleeping less effective, and you could wake up feeling tired even after sleeping for a long time.

Alcohol can also slow breathing and swell the lining of the throat, making it more difficult to breathe during sleep. This increases the likelihood of problems like snoring or sleep apnea.

If you are looking for a calming beverage, try warm milk (some research suggests that the tryptophan in milk can help speed the onset of sleep) or chamomile tea instead.

7

Cut out late-day caffeine.

Caffeine can start affecting your body in as little as 15 minutes after it is consumed. Despite the quick uptake, it can stay in your system for up to 12 hours! That's why it's particularly important to avoid caffeine in the late afternoon and evening to ensure that it will not disturb your ability to fall asleep.

You may be consuming caffeine late in the day without being aware of it. Watch out for sneakier sources of caffeine like chocolate, cola, and even decaf coffee. These all have low doses of caffeine and can affect you if you are sensitive.

Some headache medicines, weight loss pills, and pain relievers also contain caffeine. Be sure to check the labels on your products!

8

Don't starve or stuff yourself.

Take note of your pre-sleep eating habits. Being too full or hungry can negatively impact the quality of your sleep.

A large meal before bed can prompt heartburn, gas, or indigestion that will either keep you awake or wake you up later. Just lying down after a particularly large meal can cause physical discomfort.

Going to bed hungry is also a bad idea because it can wake you. If you are hungry in the evenings, try eating a light snack 1 – 2 hours before you know you will go to bed.

Avoid any foods that may cause physical discomfort. Foods with MSG are often reported to disrupt sleep, so skip the leftover Chinese takeout before bed.

9

Eat for sleep.

There's no one food that will help you slide into the perfect night's sleep, but most experts do recommend foods that contain tryptophan to help relax and calm your mind and body.

Tryptophan is processed by your body into serotonin and melatonin, both of which help regulate your sleep cycle. Eating certain foods in combination with carbohydrates helps tryptophan gain easier access to your brain where it can begin promoting sleep.

Good snack choices include a small bowl of cereal, a piece of fruit, or a piece of toast with peanut butter. If you have a sweet tooth, milk and cookies, or a small slice of apple pie with ice cream (avoid chocolate, which contains caffeine) can be a tasty, sleep-promoting snack.

10

Stop intake of fluids earlier.

As previously mentioned, alcohol can disturb your sleep, but any beverage can trigger your bladder to send your brain a wakeup signal if you drink too late in the evening.

Cut back on liquid intake after dinner. Be sure that using the restroom is on your bedtime routine.

If you have an overactive bladder and find that you rarely sleep through the night without a bathroom break, ask your doctor about potential treatment options to make you feel better and sleep well.

11

Avoid nicotine in the evening.

You might think that a cigarette will calm you down, but it can actually have a stimulating effect (similar to caffeine).

Avoid smoking before bed or in the middle of the night. In general, smoking causes less time in deep, restorative sleep. This is because the mild nicotine withdrawal that occurs during the night can cause sleep disturbances.

You may initially experience additional disturbances to your sleep if you cut back at night, but over time, sleep quality should improve as a healthy balance is restored.

12

Support a heavy head.

Did you know that your head weighs more than 10 pounds? The right pillow for you will provide the essential support you need for your neck and spine. This can help you avoid pain both at night and the following day.

A supportive pillow will maintain the slightly forward curve of your neck when you are lying down on your back. However, if your pillow is too high, the increased curvature of your neck can cause troubled breathing or snoring, which can hinder sleep. If your pillow is too soft and low, you may experience neck pain from the strain. Supportive pillows should also mold somewhat to the shape of your head to avoid unwanted pressure.

If you're shopping for a pillow upgrade, try them out in the store in order to determine which one is most comfortable for you. When you are trying out a new pillow, make sure to test it in the position that you normally sleep in.

13

A bigger bed for better sleep.

Share a bed? If you wake up in the middle of the night, your sleeping partner may be at fault.

The average, healthy sleeper moves around 15-30 times during the night. These nighttime movements also increase as we get older.

If your bed is too small or if your mattress is very sensitive to movement, you may be woken in the night by these disturbances.

If you're in the market for a new bed, choose the biggest size that will fit your budget and your bedroom. Also, look into new mattresses that are designed to minimize the transfer of movement to your partner.

Make sure both sleepers make the mattress shopping trip together so that you can get an idea of potential disturbances from anyone tossing and turning next to you.

14

Upgrade your mattress.

When was the last time you bought a new mattress? Experts advise that you should replace your mattress at least every 10 years. Although it can be pricey, your mattress is one of your most important investments.

Shop for the best value and not the lowest price! You spend about a third of your life sleeping, and your mattress can improve the quality of your sleep.

An unsupportive mattress can cause muscle stiffness, back pain, and neck pain. A mattress that is too firm can cause your limbs to fall asleep before you do!

Don't trust descriptions written by the mattress company or the salesperson. The best way to choose a mattress is to try it out. Spend time lying down on different mattresses before you make your final decision.

Finally, make sure your mattress rests on a solid foundation. Old box springs can cause your new mattress to wear out faster.

15

Limit your pet's access to your bed.

Although it might be comforting (and warm) to allow your dog or cat to sleep on your bed, it may hinder your sleep.

Just like humans, pets move in their sleep. Your dog can inadvertently wake you up. Pets can also have the habit of intentionally waking us up when they are ready to start their days.

It is unlikely that you and your pets will have the same sleep needs and he/she may decide that it is time to greet the day before your body is ready to wake up. Sleeping separately can improve the quality and duration of sleep for both of you!

16

Ban cell phones
from bed.

Disconnecting from your phone early can help you wind down, de-stress, and avoid distractions from sleep.

Make sure your phone is turned off at night if it's in your bedroom. The light or vibrations from an incoming call or message can wake you up, even if your phone is on silent.

Messages can start conversations that take away from your sleep time or prevent you from relaxing your mind before sleep. If possible, try disconnecting from technology for at least an hour before bed to avoid the stress from anxiety-arousing conversations, messages, or emails.

17

Move your clock.

Ever lie awake watching the minutes tick by, knowing you're losing more and more sleep? This can be a very stressful experience! Instead of torturing yourself, try turning your clock around or positioning it where you can't see it.

When we can't sleep, looking at the clock increases our stress levels, making it even more difficult to relax and fall asleep. Also, light from a clock can be part of the problem.

Knowing the time and how much sleep you lost won't help you when you are trying to fall back asleep!

18

Make the bed a sleep-only zone.

Our brains make associations based on what's happening around us. That's one of the reasons we can focus in environments where we regularly work.

We're conditioned to feel sleepier or more awake in certain environments. When we do work or watch TV in bed, our brains begin to associate the bedroom with these activities.

Without knowing it, you might be unintentionally conditioning yourself to feel more anxious when you see your sheets because of late nights spent finishing reports for work or paying bills in bed.

Reserve your bed for sleeping to reduce stress and sleep well!

19

Set a bedtime alarm.

Your alarm wakes you up every morning, but it can also be used to make sure you get to sleep on time every night. When you're busy, it's easy to lose track of time and miss the bedtime you intended.

If sleep doesn't feel like a priority, it can be easy to push it further and further back in time. This not only reduces the total amount of sleep time you get, but it can lead to inconsistency in bedtimes. Inconsistent bedtimes disrupt your body's ability to regulate sleep every day.

Set your alarm clock to go off at your intended bedtime every night as a reminder to get the most regular sleep possible.

20

Take a warm bath.

Many people find that a warm bath can be the perfect preparation for a good night's sleep.

Warm water can help ease your body into a more restful state and relieve stress. This helps prepare you both physically and mentally for sleep.

For even more relaxation in the tub, add in aromatherapy oils or minerals with soothing scents like chamomile, lavender, and passion flower. Low lighting, candles, and calming music can also ease you into a better night's sleep.

Stick to baths. Showers are not recommended as they can have an energizing effect.

21

Lower the thermostat.

Our internal body temperature drops as you fall asleep. You can help your body prepare for sleep by slightly lowering the external temperature.

The temperature that works best for you can range between 65 and 72 degrees.

To feel comfortable with the lower temperature, you can try wearing socks to bed. Your feet can be one of the first parts of your body to get cold.

22

Turn your bedroom into a cave.

Imagine sleeping in a cave. Try to design your bedroom to mimic this setting at night. Like a cave, your bedroom should be cool, silent, and dark.

If you live in a noisy environment, always make sure your windows are closed. Consider investing in a good pair of ear plugs or a white noise generator.

Block out as much light as possible at night. Even if it's dark when you go to bed, the early morning sun streaming in through the blinds can cause early morning wakeups.

Adjust the temperature or set the thermostat timer so you will be comfortable all night long and wake up refreshed and ready to emerge from your cave!

23

Listen to your body.

Don't force yourself to stay up if you don't have to!

When you're exhausted, you're not performing at your best. Staying up later each night causes your sleep cycle to become more and more out of sync.

If there's nothing urgent that requires your attention, your time is better spent preparing for sleep than spending an extra 30 minutes on the couch. Record that one last show and watch it tomorrow when you're refreshed.

24

Can't sleep immediately? Don't worry!

Think you should fall asleep immediately after your head hits the pillow? Think again! If you are falling asleep this fast, you are probably sleep-deprived. Make a point to schedule more sleep into your day.

Sleep should come about 15-25 minutes after you've gotten into bed. Relax and be patient. Do not get anxious if you can't fall asleep immediately – any anxiety or stress you feel will only make it more difficult to sleep.

25
Get out of bed!

If you can't fall asleep for 15-20 minutes, don't obsess over it, you'll only increase your stress level and make it even more difficult to sleep. Sometimes, the best thing to do is get up and do something else until you feel tired enough to try sleeping again.

While you are up waiting to feel sleepy, do not engage in any energizing activities or mentally taxing tasks. Do not turn on many lights when you get up, as these can make you feel even more awake. Instead, try reading a book on the couch with a low light. Return to your bed only when you feel ready to sleep again.

26

Try mental math.

Are your thoughts racing as you lie in bed?

Don't count sheep – you're likely to lose focus and concentration when doing a routine mental task like counting sheep. Instead, choose a continuous math problem that will require all of your mental focus, like counting backward from 300 by 6s.

A challenging problem will help you avoid dwelling on the anxieties and stresses of your day (or your tomorrow).

If you don't prefer math, try slowing down your thoughts by forcing yourself to say every word going through your head at a very slow pace and in a monotone voice.

27

Try these relaxation techniques.

If you're having trouble falling asleep, consider progressive muscle relaxation. Begin at your toes and work your way up your body slowly.

Starting with your toes, tense one muscle group at a time for ten seconds and then release the tension. Then, move on to the next group. If you haven't fallen asleep by the time you have completed tensing and relaxing the muscles in your face, repeat the exercise. Each full cycle should take about 25 minutes.

Focusing on your breathing can also help you ease into sleep. Follow your breathing rhythm as you inhale and exhale, paying attention to the gentle rise and fall of your abdomen.

Finally, visualizing a calming place (like a quiet seaside or country retreat) or activity can help relieve tension in your mind or body. Meditate as you drift into sleep.

28

Be careful with OTC sleep aids.

If you've ever taken an over-the-counter medication for allergies or colds, you've probably experienced the sedative effect of antihistamines.

While they might have short-term benefits for increasing sleepiness, OTC sleep aids are not advised for long-term use. Side effects like dry mouth, dizziness, and daytime drowsiness may occur. Also, antihistamine's effect can be reduced through repeated use.

Save those medications for times when you are truly sick and need them most!

29

Try a natural sleep aid.

Natural sleep aids can give you gentle benefits to improve sleep. Many natural sleep aids are safe, effective, and non-habit forming.

Typically, these supplements contain melatonin. Melatonin occurs naturally in your body and helps regulate your sleeping cycle.

Additionally, several herbal ingredients can help you get a better night's sleep. The herbs valerian and lemon balm have been used for centuries to promote relaxation and sleep. Popular in teas, the chamomile flower is commonly used to promote relaxation and sleep. Hops extract may also help reduce the amount of time required to fall asleep. Passion flower is recognized for its calming properties.

When shopping for a natural sleep aid, check for these ingredients and follow the timing and dosage instructions as written.

30

Still struggling?
Ask your doctor.

Think you're getting enough sleep, but feel exhausted all day? Experiencing sudden onsets of sleeplessness? Falling asleep at inappropriate times?

There are a number of sleep disorders and conditions that may be affecting your sleep patterns.

If you are experiencing unusual sleep disturbances, always ask your doctor about your symptoms and concerns. Many medications for unrelated conditions (including those for asthma, ADHD, hypothyroidism, depression, and more) can have an effect on your ability to fall asleep or stay asleep.

Check with your doctor or pharmacist if you experience sleep problems after starting a new medication. There may be an alternative that won't have the same impact on your sleep.

Start Sleeping Better Tonight

A night without sleep can truly feel like torture. With the knowledge, tips, and tricks you've learned in this guide, you can take control over your sleep. However, remember that change can take time. Many of the tips you've read here may require significant changes to your daily routine. Be patient - a good night's sleep is definitely worth it. Your future self will thank you for the good habits you begin today. Best wishes for a better night's sleep!